Healing and Balance Life Polycystic Ovary Syndrome

Symptoms, Causes, and Treatment Balancing Your Hormones

Copyright © 2020

All rights reserved.

DEDICATION

The author and publisher have provided this e-book to you for your personal use only. You may not make this e-book publicly available in any way. Copyright infringement is against the law. If you believe the copy of this e-book you are reading infringes on the author's copyright, please notify the publisher at: https://us.macmillan.com/piracy

Contents

Polycystic Ovary Syndrome 1

Signs You Might Have PCOS and Not Even Know It 3

Cause of Polycystic Ovary Syndrome 17

How to Manage Polycystic Ovary Syndrome 21

What to Eat If You Have PCOS 36

How Often Should PCOS Patients Go to the Doctor? 44

Polycystic Ovary Syndrome

Polycystic ovary syndrome (PCOS) is a set of symptoms due to elevated androgens in females.[4][14] Signs and symptoms of PCOS include irregular or no menstrual periods, heavy periods, excess body and facial hair, acne, pelvic pain, difficulty getting pregnant, and patches of thick, darker, velvety skin.[3] Associated conditions include type 2 diabetes, obesity, obstructive sleep apnea, heart disease, mood disorders, and endometrial cancer.[4] It is sometimes referred to as polycystic ovary disease (PCOD) when there is ultrasonographic evidence of the presence of ovarian cysts.

PCOS is due to a combination of genetic and environmental factors.[6][7][15] Risk factors include obesity, a lack of physical exercise, and a family history of someone with the condition.[8] Diagnosis is based on two of the following three findings: anovulation, high androgen levels, and ovarian cysts.[4] Cysts may be detectable by ultrasound.[9] Other conditions that produce similar symptoms include adrenal hyperplasia, hypothyroidism, and high blood levels of prolactin.[9]

PCOS has no cure as of 2020.[5] Treatment may involve lifestyle

Polycystic Ovary Syndrome

changes such as weight loss and exercise.[10][11] Birth control pills may help with improving the regularity of periods, excess hair growth, and acne.[12] Metformin and anti-androgens may also help.[12] Other typical acne treatments and hair removal techniques may be used.[12] Efforts to improve fertility include weight loss, clomiphene, or metformin.[16] In vitro fertilization is used by some in whom other measures are not effective.[16]

PCOS is the most common endocrine disorder among women between the ages of 18 and 44.[17] It affects approximately 2% to 20% of this age group depending on how it is defined.[8][13] When someone is infertile due to lack of ovulation, PCOS is the most common cause.[4] The earliest known description of what is now recognized as PCOS dates from 1721 in Italy.

Signs You Might Have PCOS and Not Even Know It

1

Darker Patches On Your Skin

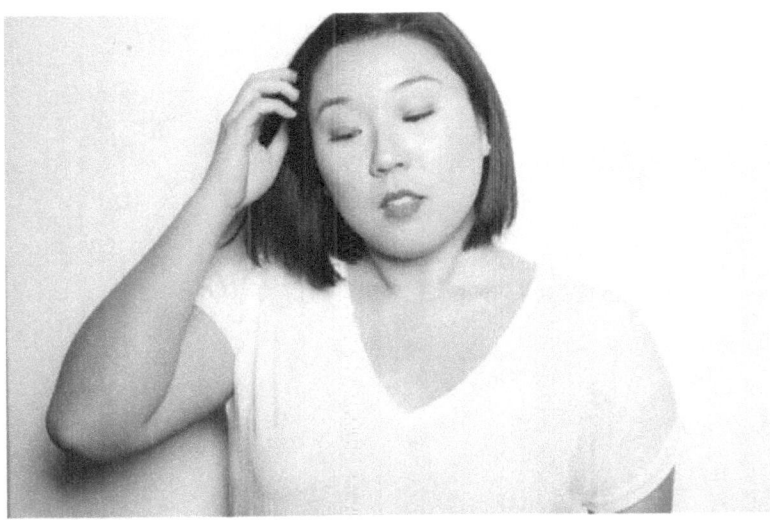

If you notice rings around your neck that are darker than your usual skin tone, it may be a sign of a shift in your hormones. "They are called acanthosis nigricans, and are most common on the back of the neck and right above the elbows," Dr. Shaughanassee Williams, DNP, CNM, founder of HealthyHER Center for Women's Care, tells Bustle. "These patches are the result of insulin resistance meaning that the woman's body has difficulty processing sugars." If you spot this change in skin tone, talk to your doctor to find out if PCOS is to blame.

2

Irregular Or Heavy Periods

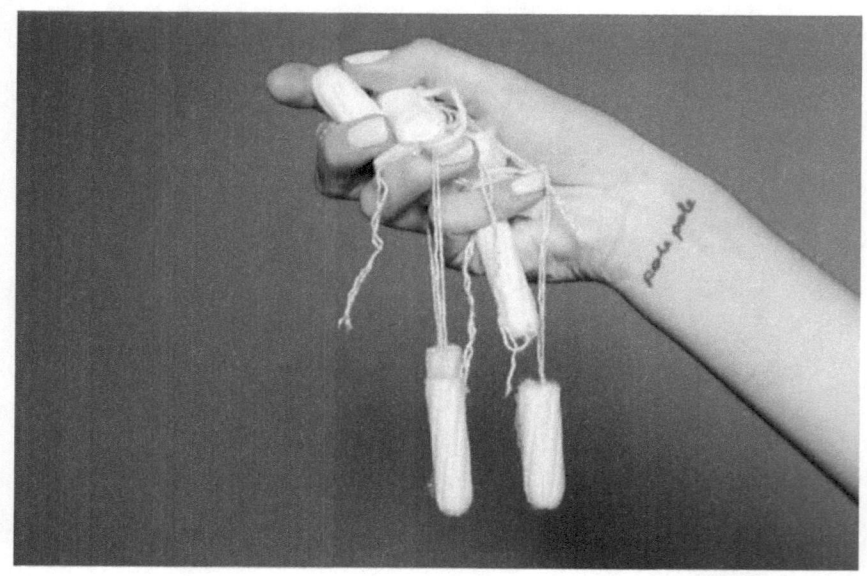

"Regardless of the diagnostic criteria that are used, [PCOS] most commonly leads to irregular periods and difficulty ovulating on a regular basis," Maria Costantini-Ferrando, MD, PhD, FACOG, at Reproductive Medicine Associates of New Jersey (RMANJ) tells Bustle.

Polycystic Ovary Syndrome

If your periods are often delayed or you have a heavy flow, talk with an OB/GYN. They can run a few tests, such as an ultrasound, to see if your irregular periods are due to PCOS.

3

Waking Up Feeling Tired

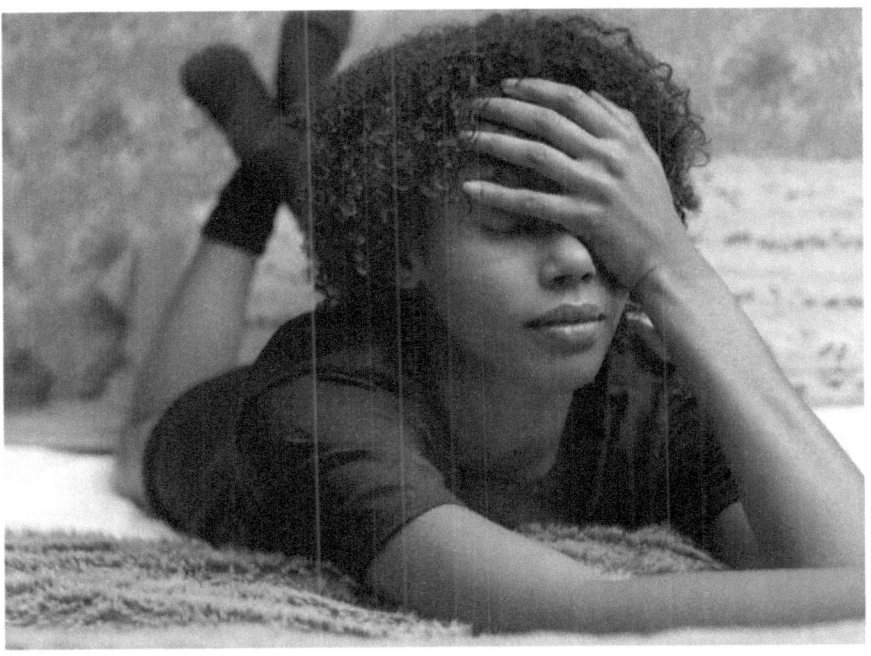

Do you tend to wake up feeling tired, despite getting those recommended seven to nine hours of shut eye? If so, it could mean you're struggling with PCOS-related symptoms during the night. As

Polycystic Ovary Syndrome

Williams says, "Sleep apnea and insomnia are two common side effects of PCOS," and both can leave you feeling exhausted.

Insomnia can make it difficult to fall asleep. And sleep apnea is a condition where your breathing is interrupted while you sleep, resulting in insufficient oxygen to your brain. Both issues have been linked to PCOS, and the resulting fatigue may help tip you off.

4

Cravings For Certain Foods

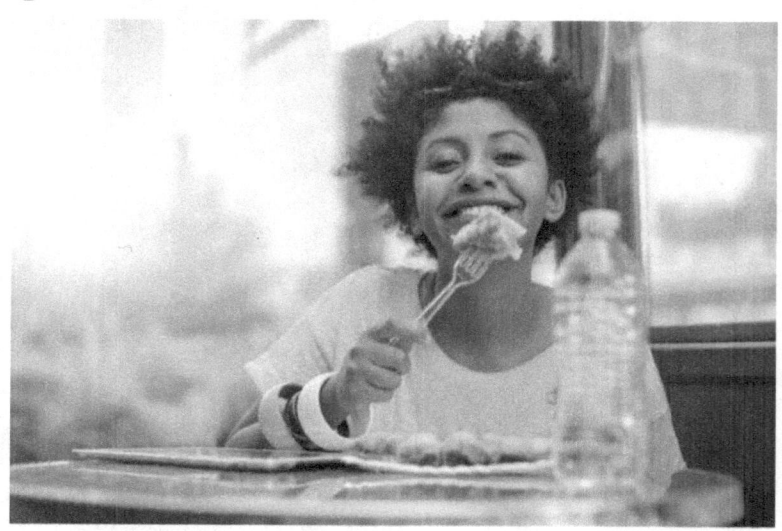

Sometimes, a craving for a certain food can be your body's way of telling you something. In the case of PCOS, you might notice that

Polycystic Ovary Syndrome

you're craving carbohydrates more often. As dietician Meghan Cichy, RDN, CEDRD, CSP, CD tells Bustle, this has a lot to do with how PCOS affects your insulin levels.

"Insulin is a hormone that acts like a key to unlock the cells of the body and enables the cells to take glucose from the bloodstream into the cell to be used as fuel," she says. "In insulin resistance, the cell 'doors' are not responding to the insulin 'key,' which leaves glucose in the blood and results in your cells starving for fuel. This can trigger cravings for carbohydrates in an attempt to take in glucose to fuel the cells." And it's why many doctors prescribe insulin medications to women who are struggling with PCOS.

5
Adult Acne

Polycystic Ovary Syndrome

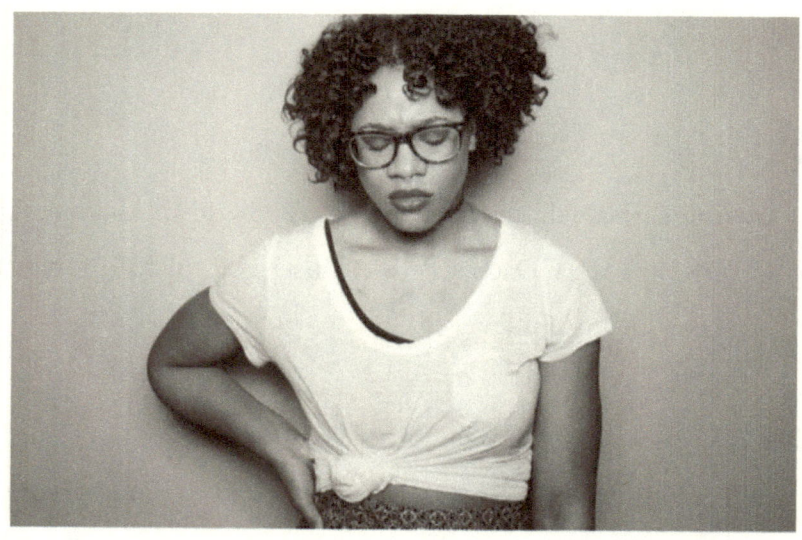

"While acne as a teen is [common], acne as an adult woman can be a sign of PCOS," Jenna McCarthy, MD, an IVFMD fertility specialist, tells Bustle. This is usually due to the hormonal changes associated with PCOS. But it can be treated, by getting to the root of the problem.

"A skin doctor or dermatologist may be the best way to avoid severe acne," Sherry Ross, MD, OB/GYN, Women's Health Expert and author of She-ology: The Definitive Guide to Women's Intimate Health. Period, tells Bustle. "Anti-androgens [decreasing testosterone], antibiotics, and special medicated skin washes are also used to keep the acne under control."

Polycystic Ovary Syndrome

6

Trouble Conceiving

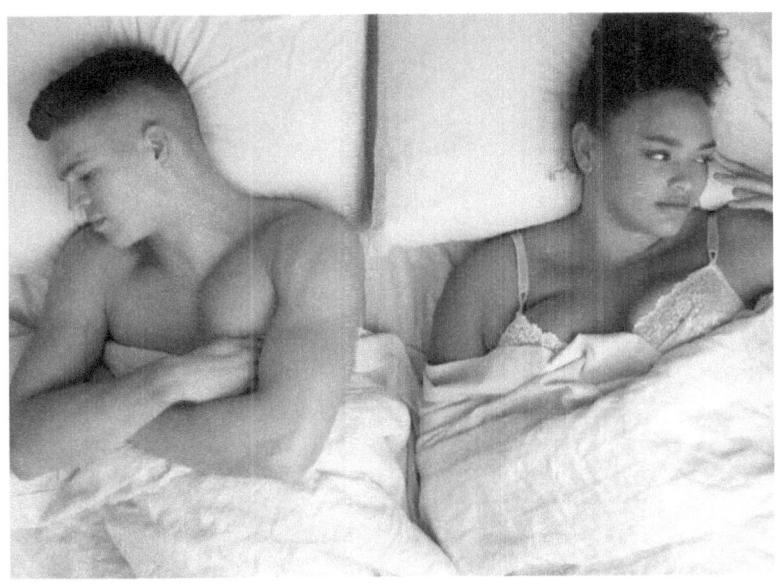

Another subtle thing to watch out for? Unpredictable ovulation tests. If you're trying to become pregnant, and would like to map out your ovulation dates with an at-home kit, you might notice that you can't seem to get a positive result.

"If someone is trying to conceive, she may also have difficulties interpreting any ovulation prediction kits because sometimes, they never get a positive or every day says it's positive," Dr. Erika Munch,

Polycystic Ovary Syndrome

a reproductive endocrinologist at Texas Fertility Center, tells Bustle. "And both outcomes are very frustrating."

If this is happening to you, PCOS may be what's messing up your hormones, and thus messing up your ovulation test results. And since experts have linked PCOS to infertility, speaking with a doctor ASAP will be in your best interest, if you're trying to conceive.

7

Thinning Hair

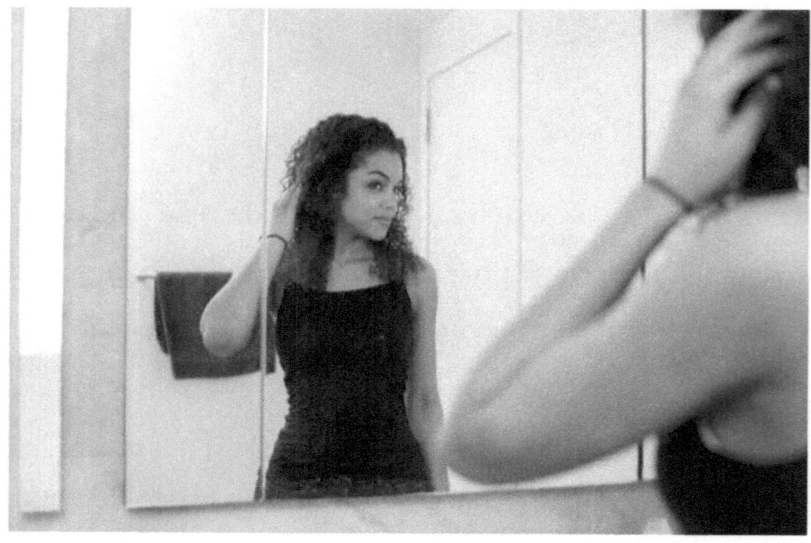

While it's common to lose up to 100 strands of hair a day, take note if it seems like your hair is thinning — especially if you can see more of your scalp than usual. As Williams says, thinning hair might be due to excess testosterone in the body, which "can cause women to have a condition similar to male-pattern baldness." But if this is happening to you, do not panic — talking with your OB/GYN about a potential PCOS diagnosis can help get to the root of this problem, and treat it.

8

Hair In New Places

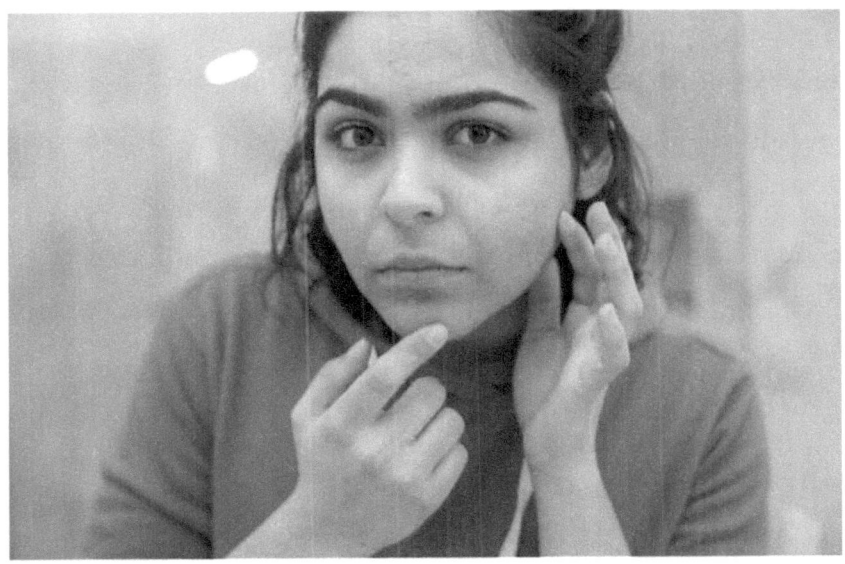

While everyone has different levels of hair growth on their body, sometimes new patches of hair can be a sign of a hormonal imbalance. "Many women with PCOS have increased effects of the male hormones we all have, because the body hasn't made enough protein to help bind these extra male hormones," says Munch. "For some women, that can mean hair in places ... like the lip, chin, sideburns ... or problems with acne."

The hair itself isn't the issue nor is it anything to be ashamed of, but the reason behind it can be cause for concern, in some instances. Since PCOS can affect your health, it's a good idea to pay attention to little clues like this from your body, and talk with a doctor to make sure your hormones are properly balanced.

9

Anxiety and Depression

Polycystic Ovary Syndrome

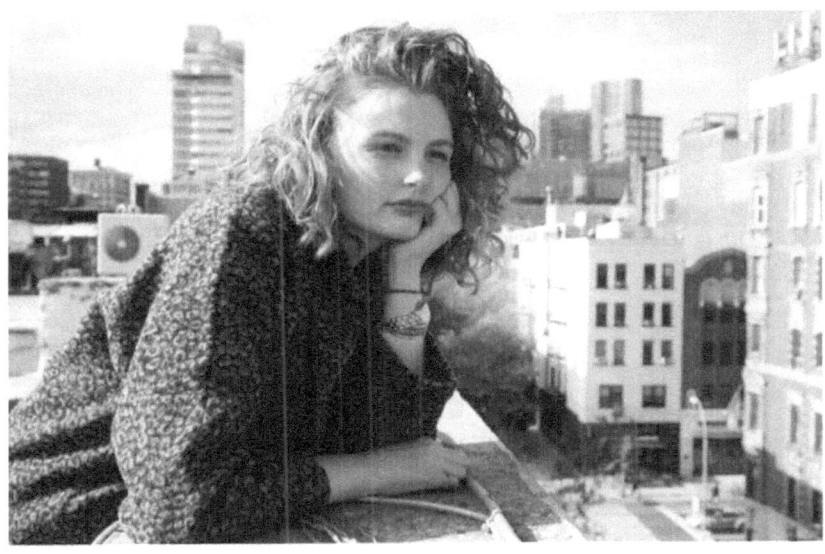

According to Ross, anxiety and depression can be a sign of PCOS. So if you haven't been feeling like yourself and can't quite figure out why, a trip to an OB/GYN should be on your list of things to do.

Of course, there are many factors at play when it comes to mental health, but sometimes an underlying health issue, like PCOS can make you feel worse, especially since it can impact your hormones. If you feel that you are struggling with anxiety or depression, confiding in a doctor, therapist, or loved one can guide you toward the help you need to feel well again.

10

Unexplained Health Issues, Like High Blood Pressure

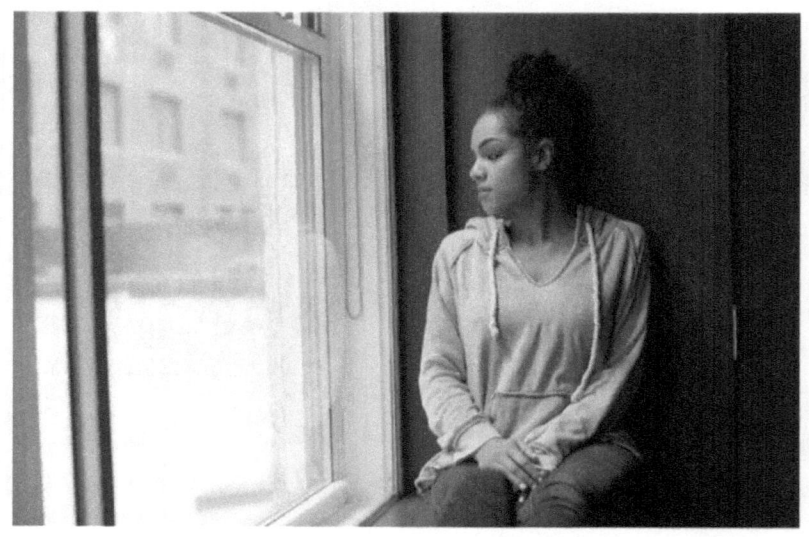

You might not immediately think of PCOS as the cause of your anxiety and depression, but both have be linked linked to the disorder. And so are many other health concerns. As Ross says, "The list is long and includes ... heart attacks, high blood pressure, high cholesterol ... endometrial cancer, and sleep apnea." Although some of these conditions are extreme, and represent worst case scenario situations, being mindful of your health and speaking with your doctor if you experience any changes can help treat the issue early.

11

Diabetes

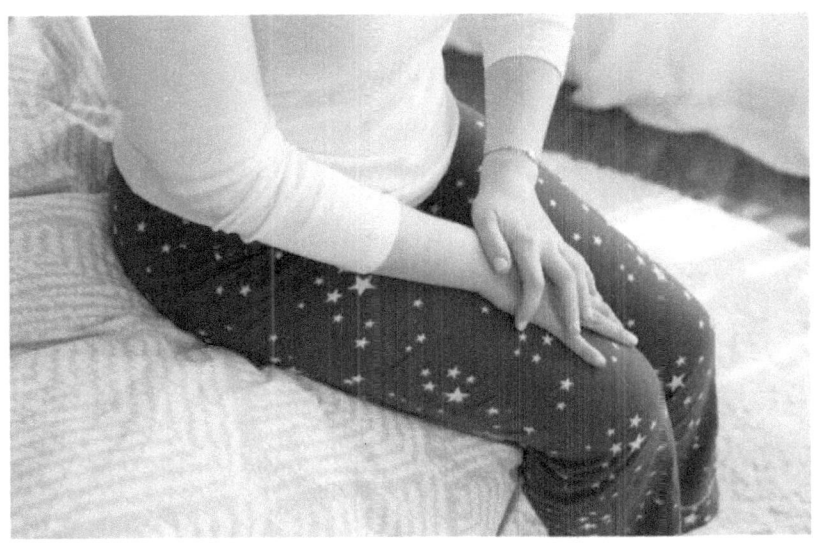

If you've been diagnosed with pre-diabetes or diabetes, it may be a good idea to be checked for PCOS, too. "Women with PCOS may ... become less efficient at processing sugars (glucose and carbohydrates) from their diets. As a result, women can also develop glucose intolerance (pre diabetic state) or resistance to the insulin that their body makes," Dr. Aaron Styer, Medical Director with CCRM Boston tells Bustle. "This can result in ... the development of diabetes, increased cholesterol levels, and an increased risks of heart attack and stroke later in life. As a result, women with PCOS should be screened for diabetes and abnormal cholesterol levels during their initial evaluation to reduce the risk of complications later in life."

But there is no need to fret — if you think you might have polycystic ovary syndrome, check in with your doctor. They can check to see if the symptoms mentioned above are, in fact, due to PCOS. And then prescribe you a treatment plan, so you can start feeling better.

Cause of Polycystic Ovary Syndrome

PCOS is a heterogeneous disorder of uncertain cause.[26][27] There is some evidence that it is a genetic disease. Such evidence includes the familial clustering of cases, greater concordance in monozygotic compared with dizygotic twins and heritability of endocrine and metabolic features of PCOS.[7][26][27] There is some evidence that exposure to higher than typical levels of androgens and the anti-Müllerian hormone (AMH) in utero increases the risk of developing PCOS in later life.[28]

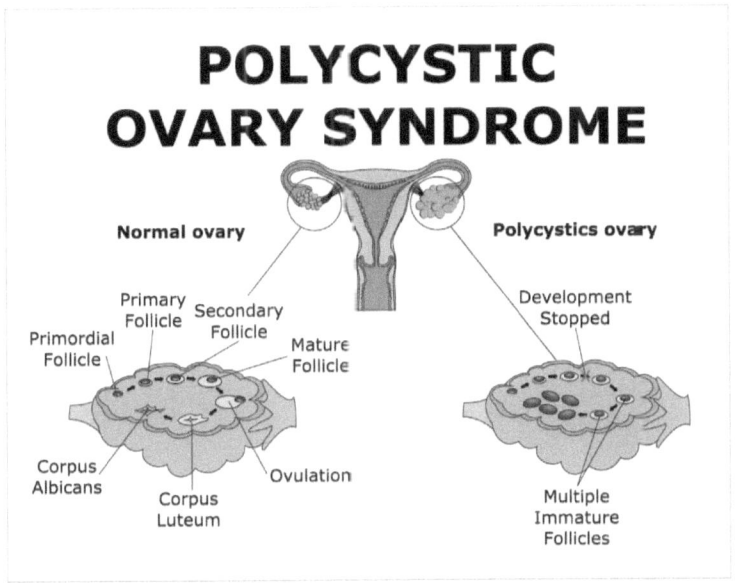

Polycystic Ovary Syndrome

Genetics

The genetic component appears to be inherited in an autosomal dominant fashion with high genetic penetrance but variable expressivity in females; this means that each child has a 50% chance of inheriting the predisposing genetic variant(s) from a parent, and, if a daughter receives the variant(s), the daughter will have the disease to some extent.[27][29][30][31] The genetic variant(s) can be inherited from either the father or the mother, and can be passed along to both sons (who may be asymptomatic carriers or may have symptoms such as early baldness and/or excessive hair) and daughters, who will show signs of PCOS.[29][31] The phenotype appears to manifest itself at least partially via heightened androgen levels secreted by ovarian follicle theca cells from women with the allele.[30] The exact gene affected has not yet been identified.[7][27][32] In rare instances, single-gene mutations can give rise to the phenotype of the syndrome.[33] Current understanding of the pathogenesis of the syndrome suggests, however, that it is a complex multigenic disorder.[34]

The severity of PCOS symptoms appears to be largely determined by factors such as obesity.[7][17][35] PCOS has some aspects of a

Polycystic Ovary Syndrome

metabolic disorder, since its symptoms are partly reversible. Even though considered as a gynecological problem, PCOS consists of 28 clinical symptoms.[citation needed]

Even though the name suggests that the ovaries are central to disease pathology, cysts are a symptom instead of the cause of the disease. Some symptoms of PCOS will persist even if both ovaries are removed; the disease can appear even if cysts are absent. Since its first description by Stein and Leventhal in 1935, the criteria of diagnosis, symptoms, and causative factors are subject to debate. Gynecologists often see it as a gynecological problem, with the ovaries being the primary organ affected. However, recent insights show a multisystem disorder, with the primary problem lying in hormonal regulation in the hypothalamus, with the involvement of many organs. The name PCOD is used when there is ultrasonographic evidence. The term PCOS is used due to the fact that there is a wide spectrum of symptoms possible, and cysts in the ovaries are seen only in 15% of people.[36]

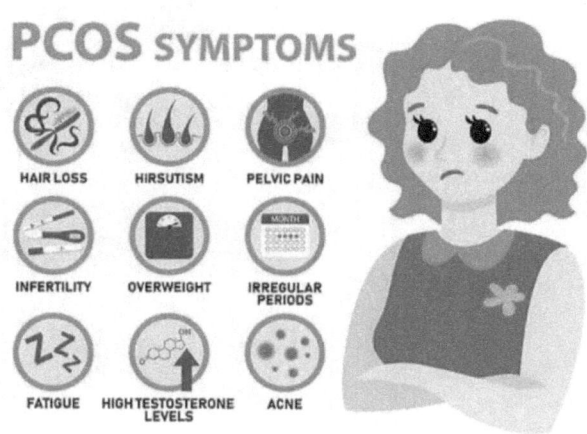

Environment

PCOS may be related to or worsened by exposures during the prenatal period, epigenetic factors, environmental impacts (especially industrial endocrine disruptors,[37] such as bisphenol A and certain drugs) and the increasing rates of obesity

How to Manage Polycystic Ovary Syndrome

Method

1

Maintaining a Healthy Weight

1

Set a reasonable goal for weight loss. Losing weight is often recommended for women who are diagnosed with PCOS. However, you do not need to lose a ton of weight to see improvements in your condition. Even losing 10% of your body weight may help to correct the hormonal issues that are causing your PCOS.[2]

For example, if you weigh 250 pounds, then try setting a goal to lose 25 pounds over the course of five months. This is a five pound weight loss per month, which will mean that you will need to lose one to two pounds per week. This is a reasonable, healthy weight loss rate.

Polycystic Ovary Syndrome

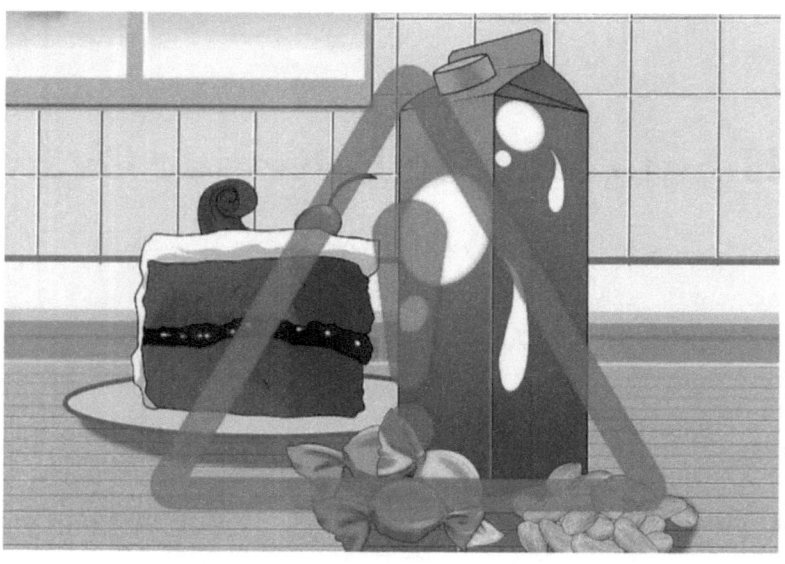
2

Control insulin by cutting out sweets and carbs. Those with polycystic ovary syndrome experience increased insulin levels. Insulin is a hormone, and when more of it is present, people feel hungrier sooner and more often, which causes them to eat more and gain weight. It is crucial for those with polycystic ovary syndrome to regulate their weight to avoid the most severe symptoms. [3]

Eliminate sweet treats. Most of us enjoy a sweet piece of cake, candy, bread, or pie at least every now and then. Sometimes, it feels difficult to go a day without having some chocolate or cookies. However, the more sugar you eat, the more insulin you will produce. Eat fresh fruit when you need your fix.

Cut down on carbohydrates. Food like white pasta, white bread, potatoes and corn tastes good and can be comforting to eat, but it also heightens insulin levels. Consume multigrain bread, vegetables, or whole wheat pasta instead of high glycemic foods.

Stop drinking soda and other sugary drinks. Pepsi might be your drink of choice, but soft drinks are filled with sugar. Even healthier seeming options like juice contain too much sugar. Choose plain water, water flavored with strawberry or cucumber, seltzer water, or unsweetened ice tea.[4] However, do not switch to diet soda to solve this problem. People who drink diet soda tend to weigh more and consume more calories from solid foods.[5]

3

Help yourself to more protein. To help block insulin and to keep your weight on track, eat more meat and legumes. Healthy sources of protein are a good choice when you need a snack, and you should consume protein at every meal. Just don't go overboard

Prioritize protein. Eating protein-filled food helps fill us up and provides energy. Eating items like peanut butter and other nuts, fish, chicken, pork, red meat, eggs, beans (black beans, lentils, lima beans, etc), and soy counteracts insulin produced by eating other food. Sustaining a more protein-based diet can help you maintain a healthier weight. [6]

Consider portion size. After you change your diet, you still have to be aware of how much you eat. Clearly, savoring a 16-ounce steak or three servings of fried fish during Friday dinners won't help you keep your weight down. It is better to eat smaller portions throughout the day. [7]

Read the labels. Sometimes, it might seem like our food choices are healthy, but they aren't. Be aware of how much sodium and sugar are in the food that you eat. Use a fit bit or buy a calorie counter to help you in this endeavor.

Polycystic Ovary Syndrome

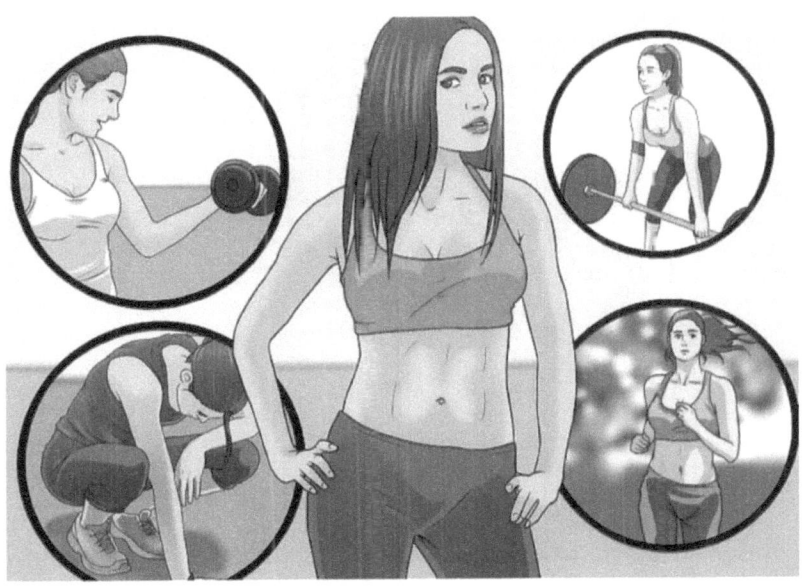

4

Exercise regularly. Exercising boosts the heart rate and helps us lose weight. It can also alleviate PMS symptoms or feelings of anxiety, which also come along with polycystic ovary syndrome. Women with this illness can benefit especially from exercising right after they eat. Figure out what kind of exercise is enjoyable for you and build it into your routine. [8]

Using exercise equipment is one option. You can go to the gym and use an elliptical machine, lift weights, ride a stationary bike, and more. If you have a machine at home, that is even more convenient.

Another option is to hike outdoors, which can be more enjoyable for those who like to breathe in the fresh air. Even big cities offer large, wooded parks, so seek out a pleasurable environment! While walking trails, you might see interesting wildlife, too!

Playing sports can be fun and definitely helps burn calories. You don't have to be a pro; sign up for a community kickball or softball league. Get that blood flowing and beat down those insulin levels.

Yoga and pilates are other great forms of exercise. The stretching and breathing exercises relax you and help sustain a normal weight. These exercises also strengthen your muscles.

You can join a zumba, hip hop, step aerobics, kickboxing or similar class. These are great choices for those who like to dance. You'll boost your cardio and have a blast doing so.

Method 2

Dealing With Irregular Periods, Infertility and Excess Hair

Polycystic Ovary Syndrome

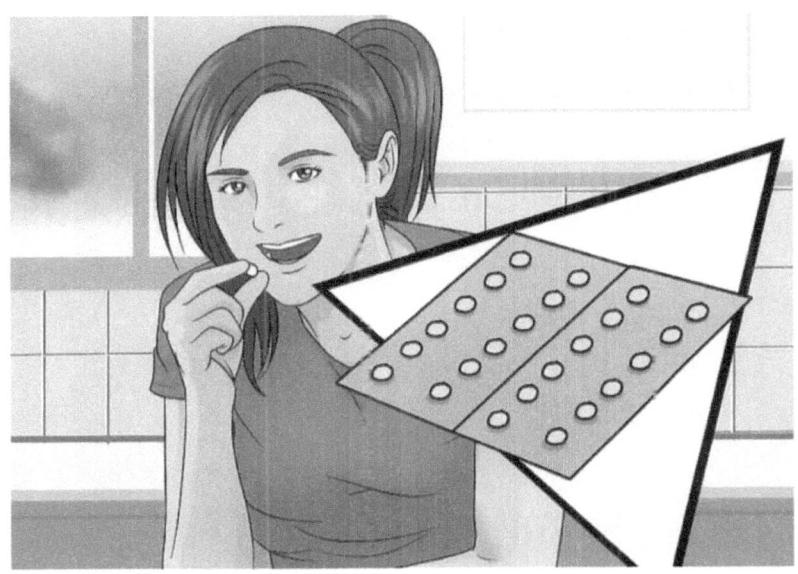

1

Take birth control pills or progesterone to manage your period. When your period interferes with your daily life, take action. One common method is to use birth control pills. The different dosages of hormones that they contain can help balance out problems with your hormones. Using progesterone is an alternative that will give similar results for those who do not like birth control pills.[9]

Remember to take your birth control pills every day at the same time. If you accidentally skip a dose, do what the directions say.

Administer progesterone as directed by your doctor. You will usually take it for only ten to fourteen days per month. Ask to try a different length of time if it doesn't seem to work. [10]

Be patient when starting these treatments. It will take several months to figure out if they will have positive effects. If you experience severe effects listed as possibilities in the informational brochure, contact your doctor immediately.

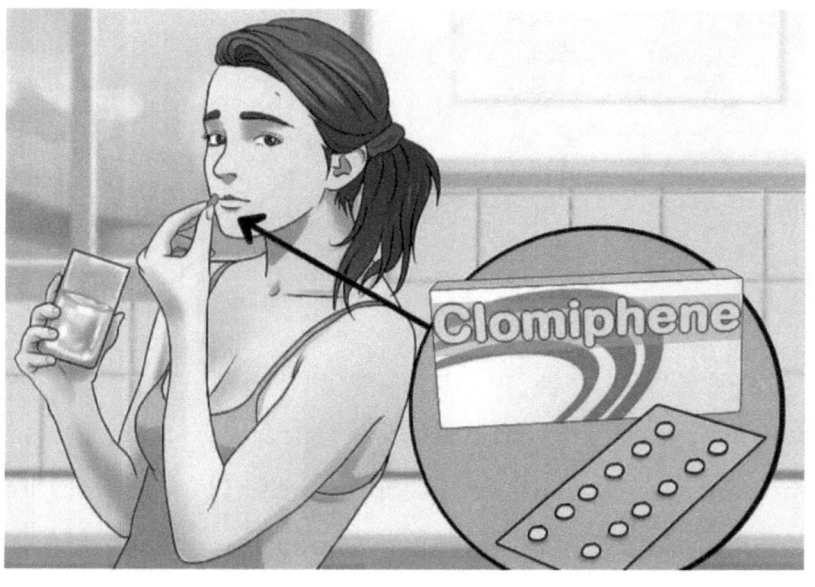

2

Use Clomiphene or other hormonal medicine to address infertility. If you desire to start a family but have not been able to conceive, it might because you are not ovulating properly. The illness prevents ovarian follicles from maturing and producing eggs.[11] Clomiphene or similar medications can spur ovulation. [12]

Polycystic Ovary Syndrome

You can try metformin alongside the Clomiphene if Clomiphene does not produce results. [13]

There are alternatives to Clomiphene if it doesn't work. Your doctor might prescribe follicle-stimulating hormone (FSH) and luteinizing hormone (LH) medications. They usually come as injections. [14]

As always, you should follow your doctor's recommendations during this time to avoid complications.

3

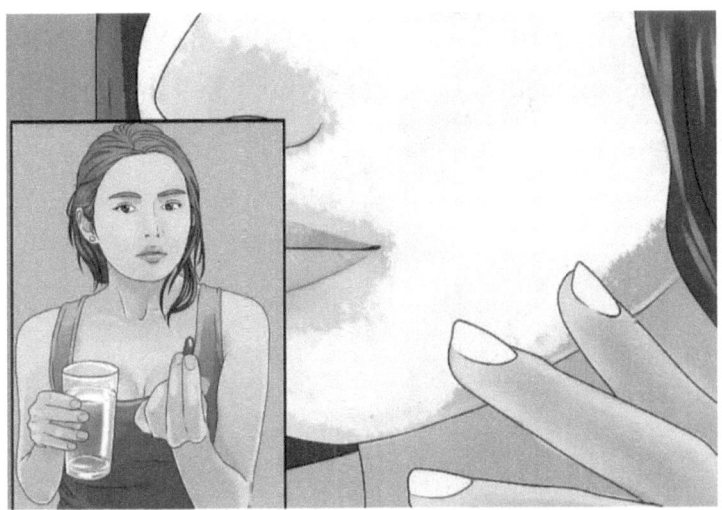

Try facial masks or medication for unwanted hair. As a woman, having excess hair is not pleasant to deal with. If constantly shaving or using fading creams becomes a hassle, administering these treatments can help. [15]

You can make a face mask with turmeric or eggs to apply to your face. Turmeric is antibacterial and it can stop hair growth. You just need to blend it with equal parts flour and some water. Mixing an egg white with a half tablespoon of corn starch and tablespoon of sugar has a similar effect. [16]

Using the drugs Aldactone or Vaniqa will lessen the amount of androgen that your body produces, which will result in less hair growth. [17]

You have to use contraception while using medication because spironolactone, an active ingredient, can result in birth defects in children.

Polycystic Ovary Syndrome

4

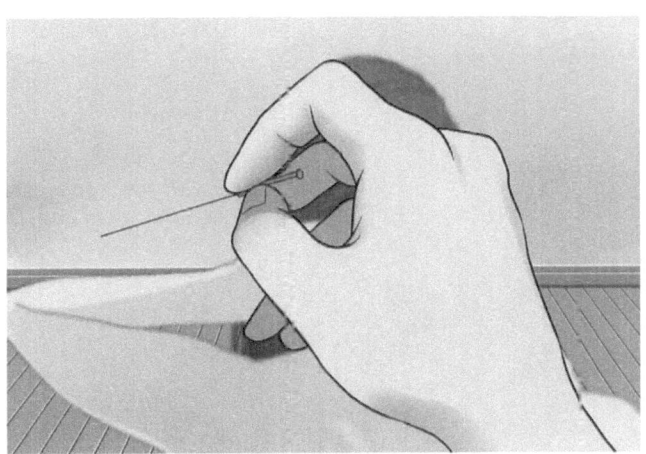

Get acupuncture. This ancient Chinese practice has documented beneficial uses. It focuses on tapping into the energy found in your body's pathways. For women with polycystic ovary syndrome, acupuncture takes place near knee, lower back and lower belly to stimulate the ovaries. [18]

Certain forms of acupuncture can work as well as or better than traditional medicine.

Acupuncture can actually help balance your hormones.[19]

Testosterone levels will decrease, the menstrual cycle might regulate, and ovulation may improve. [20]

Thousands of women have used it and have experienced positive results. [21]

Method

3

Staying Positive

1

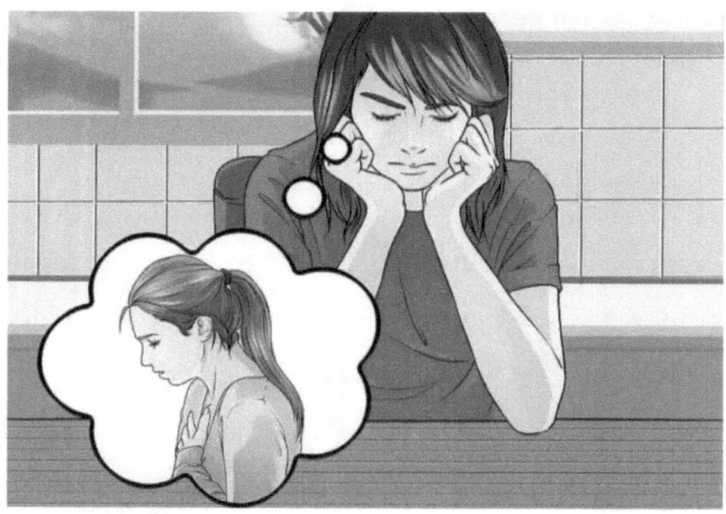

Practice radical acceptance. Sometimes we become angry when we realize that we can not control something in our lives, like our bodies. Often, we might rebel by doing exactly what we are not supposed to. Instead, we have to accept our circumstances to stay healthy. [22]

Don't deny that you have an illness. In order to live a productive life, you must be realistic about your situation. [23]

Remind yourself daily that you are not alone. [24]

Polycystic Ovary Syndrome

Educate yourself about the illness. Being informed benefits us mentally and emotionally--ignorance is not bliss when it comes to a serious health concern. [25]

2

Join a support group. Groups for women who have polycystic ovary syndrome exist. Look online to find a group in your area and attend a meeting or two. Making connections with others has many benefits. [26]

You will feel better after sharing your experiences, especially if you don't already know someone else who has the syndrome.

You can also learn a lot from talking with like-minded people, like other tips for treating symptoms.

Strangers are usually be more objective than close friends or family members. You shouldn't have to worry about judgment while at a support group meeting.

Polycystic Ovary Syndrome

3

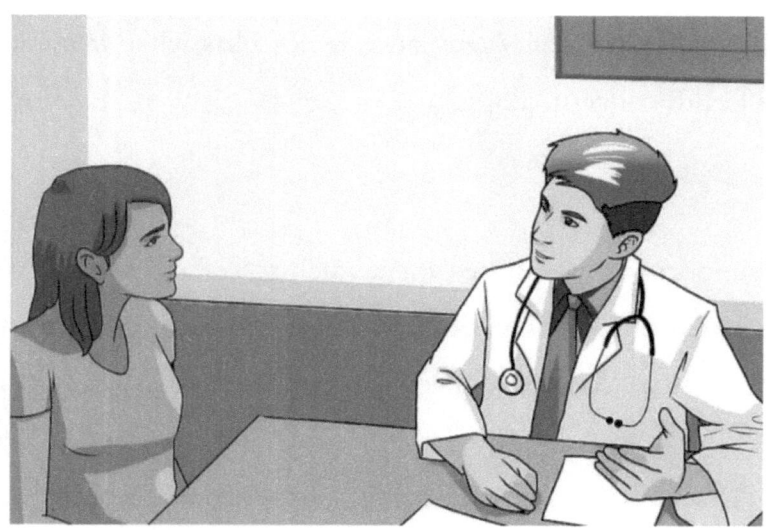

Seek counseling. If you are a private person, seeing a personal counselor is another option. People use therapy for many different reasons. Counseling can be especially helpful for women who experience fertility issues. [27]

No audience of strangers will be in the room, listening and looking. This is a plus for those who might feel uncomfortable attending a support group.

You can vent about how you are feeling about having polycystic ovary syndrome.

If you are not sure how to deal with the illness, a counselor can help you formulate an action plan.

4

Learn to meditate. After being diagnosed with polycystic ovary syndrome, it is important to reduce stressful feelings as much as possible. [28] Meditation involves breathing deeply, being mindful of the moment, and blocking out negative or chaotic thoughts.

The most useful benefit of meditation is that it will lessen your anxiety. [29]

You will also discover new solutions to pressing concerns. Sometimes we think about things in only one way, which puts us in a rut.

It will be easier for you to conquer pessimistic feelings and feel more upbeat

What to Eat If You Have PCOS

Two of the primary ways that diet affects PCOS are weight management and insulin production and resistance.

However, insulin plays a significant role in PCOS, so managing insulin levels with a PCOS diet is one of the best steps people can take to manage the condition.

Many people with PCOS have insulin resistance. In fact, more than 50 percent of those with PCOS develop diabetes or pre-diabetes before the age of 40. Diabetes is directly related to how the body processes insulin.

Following a diet that meets a person's nutritional needs, maintains a healthy weight, and promotes good insulin levels can help people with PCOS feel better.

Polycystic Ovary Syndrome

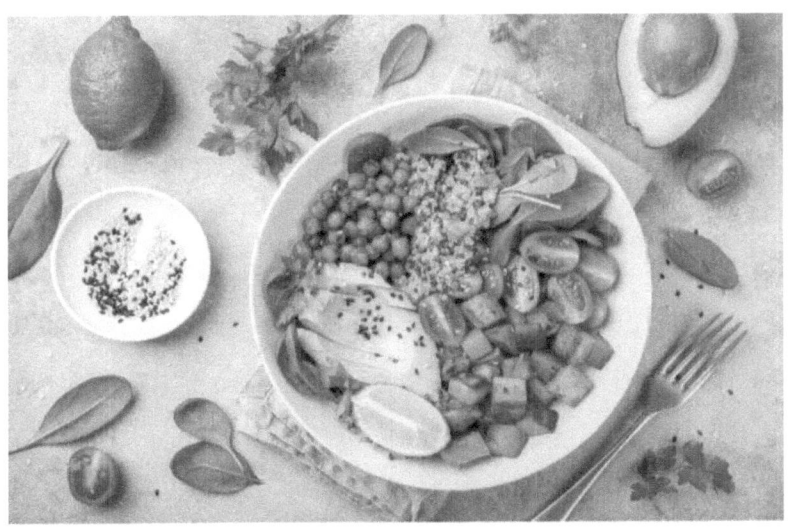

Foods to eat

Research has found that what people eat has a significant effect on PCOS. That said, there is currently no standard diet for PCOS.

However, there is widespread agreement about which foods are beneficial and seem to help people manage their condition, and which foods to avoid.

Three diets that may help people with PCOS manage their symptoms are:

- A low glycemic index (GI) diet: The body digests foods with a low GI more slowly, meaning they do not cause insulin levels to rise as much or as quickly as other foods, such as some carbohydrates. Foods in a low GI diet include whole grains, legumes, nuts, seeds, fruits, starchy vegetables, and other unprocessed, low-carbohydrate foods.

- An anti-inflammatory diet: Anti-inflammatory foods, such as berries, fatty fish, leafy greens, and extra virgin olive oil, may reduce inflammation-related symptoms, such as fatigue.
- The DASH diet: Doctors often recommend the Dietary Approaches to Stop Hypertension (DASH) diet to reduce the risk or impact of heart disease. It may also help manage PCOS symptoms. A DASH diet is rich in fish, poultry, fruits, vegetables whole grain, and low-fat dairy produce. The diet discourages foods that are high in saturated fat and sugar.

A 2015 study found that obese women who followed a specially-designed DASH diet for 8 weeks saw a reduction in insulin resistance and belly fat compared to those that did not follow the same diet.

Polycystic Ovary Syndrome

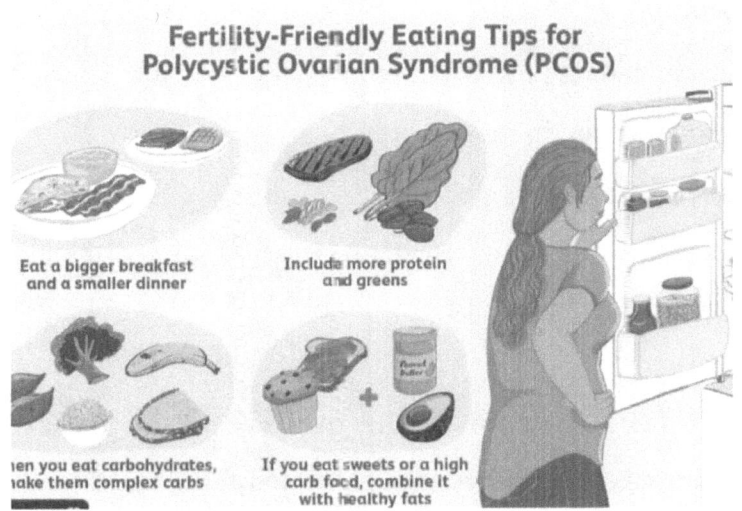

A healthful PCOS diet can also include the following foods:

- natural, unprocessed foods
- high-fiber foods
- fatty fish, including salmon, tuna, sardines, and mackerel
- kale, spinach, and other dark, leafy greens
- dark red fruits, such as red grapes, blueberries, blackberries, and cherries
- broccoli and cauliflower
- dried beans, lentils, and other legumes
- healthful fats, such as olive oil, as well as avocados and

coconuts
- nuts, including pine nuts, walnuts, almonds, and pistachios
- dark chocolate in moderation
- spices, such as turmeric and cinnamon

Researchers looking at a range of healthful diet plans found the following slight differences. For example:

- Individuals lost more weight with a diet emphasizing monounsaturated fats rather than saturated fats. An example of this kind of diet is the anti-inflammatory diet, which encourages people to eat plant-based fats, such as olive and other vegetable oils.
- People who followed a low-carbohydrate or a low-GI diet saw improved insulin metabolism and lower cholesterol levels. People with PCOS who followed a low-GI diet also reported a better quality of life and more regular periods.

In general, studies have found that losing weight helps women with PCOS, regardless of which specific kind of diet they follow.

Polycystic Ovary Syndrome

Foods to avoid

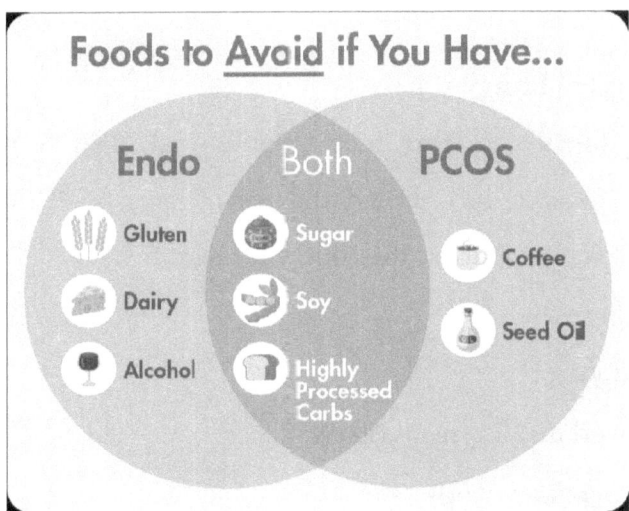

In general, people on a PCOS diet should avoid foods already widely seen as unhealthful. These include:

- Refined carbohydrates, such as mass-produced pastries and white bread.
- Fried foods, such as fast food.
- Sugary beverages, such as sodas and energy drinks.
- Processed meats, such as hot dogs, sausages, and luncheon meats.
- Solid fats, including margarine, shortening, and lard.

- Excess red meat, such as steaks, hamburgers, and pork.

Other lifestyle changes

Lifestyle changes can also help people with PCOS manage the condition. Research has shown that combining a PCOS diet with physical activity can lead to the following benefits:

- weight loss
- improved insulin metabolism
- more regular periods
- reduced levels of male hormones and male-pattern hair growth
- lower cholesterol levels

Studies have also found that behavioral strategies can help women achieve the weight management goals that, in turn, help manage PCOS symptoms. These practices include:

- goal-setting
- social support networks
- self-monitoring techniques
- caring for psychological well-being

Polycystic Ovary Syndrome

Reducing stress through self-care practices, such as getting enough sleep, avoiding over-commitment, and making time to relax, can also help a person manage PCOS.

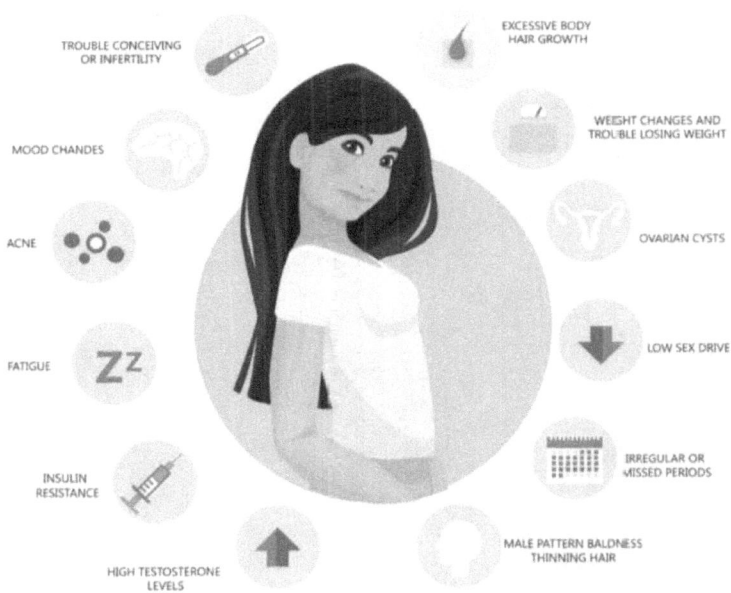

How Often Should PCOS Patients Go to the Doctor?

If issues come up way in advance of your next appointment, don't hesitate to call the office or schedule a visit. It's better to handle concerns promptly in case something more serious is going on. As always, make sure to follow the advice of your doctor, and keep the recommended schedule for routine appointments and other testing. Here's a look at the different doctors that may be a part of your healthcare team.

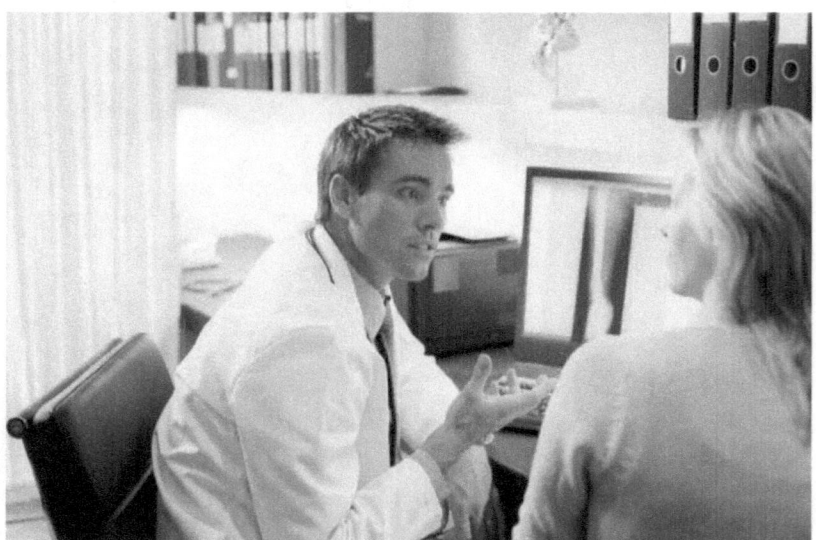

Primary Care Physician
If you are healthy and don't have any chronic medical conditions like

Polycystic Ovary Syndrome

diabetes, visiting your primary care physician, or PCP, once a year should be sufficient. Due to the risk of developing complications from PCOS, though, it's important to see your PCP annual for a physical.

Your yearly visit should include testing your blood pressure, cholesterol, and blood sugar levels.2 If any of these are abnormal, further testing, or more frequent visits, may be warranted.

It's also possible that the doctor may ask you to monitor yourself at home, as is most commonly done with high blood pressure and diabetes. Make sure you understand the instructions, including how often and when to test, and what you should do if you have abnormal results. It can also be helpful to keep a written log with your results that you can show the doctor at your next visit.

Polycystic Ovary Syndrome

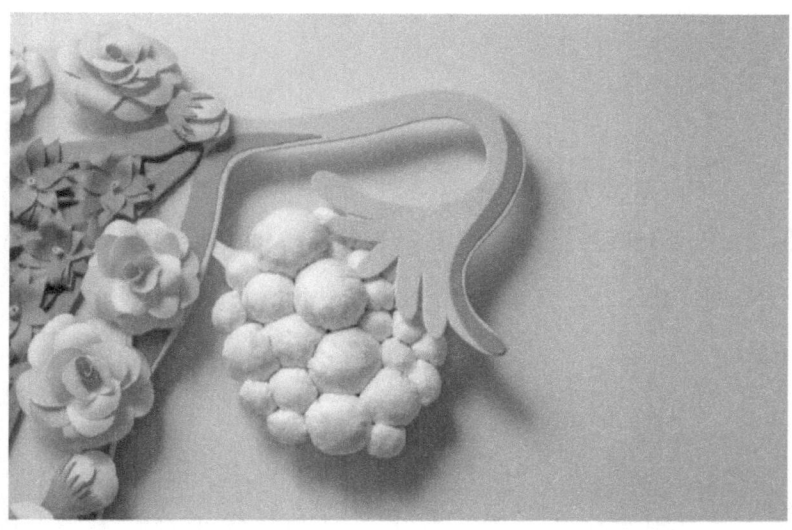

Ob/Gyn

If you're having regular periods or are on the pill, you shouldn't need to see a gynecologist any more frequently than if you didn't have PCOS. Be sure to keep your annual check-ups for a pap smear, clinical breast exam and whatever other testing the doctor recommends.

Women with PCOS are at a slightly higher risk of developing endometrial cancer: the risk increases the fewer periods a woman has.3 Each month, the uterine lining thickens in anticipation of pregnancy, and certain hormonal changes occur throughout the cycle to cause ovulation (the release of an egg from the ovary). If a fertilized egg is not implanted in the uterus, the body sheds the lining about two weeks after ovulation occurs, and the whole process restarts the next month.

Women with PCOS do not always ovulate regularly, causing the uterine lining to become exposed to higher than usual amounts of estrogen. The lining becomes thicker than normal, potentially causing cancer cells to begin growing.

The risk of endometrial cancer is significantly diminished when you're on the birth control pill, even if you don't get regular periods.4 The pill prevents your uterine lining from building up and regulates your hormones. If you're getting fewer than 8 or 9 periods a year and you aren't on the birth control pill, it's important to make an appointment to see your ob/gyn soon.5

Endocrinologist
If you are under the care of an endocrinologist and your PCOS symptoms are under control, your doctor will likely want to see you only once a year.

Polycystic Ovary Syndrome

Basic hormonal levels should be checked annually, as well as your blood sugar levels, blood pressure, and cholesterol.2 If any testing is abnormal, your doctor may send you for follow-up testing with a cardiologist (heart specialist).

Make sure to verify with your doctor when you should plan to follow up, and whether any testing should be done before that visit.

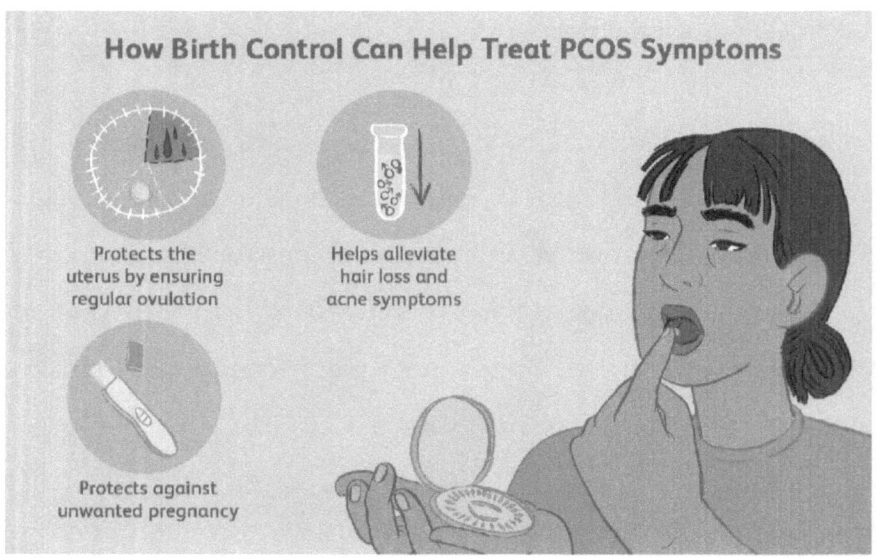

Fertility Specialist

Undergoing fertility treatment is completely different from seeing other specialists. Pursuing fertility treatment requires multiple visits, sometimes even several times a week. It's extremely important to keep those appointments, especially the daily monitoring ones.

While it may seem easy to slack off and miss a visit or two, crucial medication changes can be necessary, and missing those appointments may cause those changes to be missed.

Make sure that you understand exactly what follow-up is required, and when. Using a calendar, (either paper or digital) is instrumental in keeping track of all those appointments.

www.ingramcontent.com/pod-product-compliance
Lightning Source LLC
Chambersburg PA
CBHW030514220526
45464CB00006B/2788